# EATING YELLOW

# EATING YELLOW

Florence Duff-Scott

ISBN 978-1-914278-11-2

*This edition has been published in support of Central London Samaritans*

Photographs © Florence Duff-Scott
Cover images © Florence Duff-Scott
Foreword © Lisa St Aubin de Terán

Cover, book design and editing by Albarrojo
Published by Amaurea Press

Amaurea Press is an imprint of Amaurea Creative Productions Ltd., London, United Kingdom
www.amaurea.co.uk

*For JoJo*

# Contents

# Foreword

Dear Florence,

We used to be so close: too close, some said. But can two people who love each other be too close? That is, until something happened in Amsterdam. Not a specific something, more a drifting apart while you opened your heart to others. You the socialite: the butterfly. To flit. To flirt.

'And so talented! Have you heard her sing?'

'Have you seen her paint? And she writes her own songs? And makes her own lasagne.'

I knew some of those lovers; but others were strangers – rumoured ones with names I didn't know; although they were names you probably whispered in your sleep. Did you love them? Do you miss them? Did they know how fragile you were under your perfect mask?

You acted happy, but what did it feel like to be smothered by love? What does it feel like to have been lost for so many years and then to find yourself? I wonder too, could you hear your voice inside your head before it escaped? And was it your voice that escaped or was it you? And escaped from what? From whom? From being tormented? From tormenting yourself?

I still have a photo of you looking so petite in a blue-striped dress against a huge stone wall in Italy: feeling your way along it carefully because before you embraced recklessness you were always cautious.

'And as pretty as a porcelain doll.'

Petted and feted and too sweet for anyone (or for me, at least) to see your rage gathering. There is no point in being too sweet. Sugar kills. And there is no point in rage. Rage kills.

Analyze this and analyze that, or live for the now and be you as you are and not as I or anyone would see you or have you be.

You have found your voice now and can say 'I am' and 'I am' and be.

You seemed to be trapped in a paradox: embracing danger like an old friend, teetering on the brink for the thrill of it until you found your own way out of the darkness. That took courage.

Not long ago the threads inside you unravelled, you studied them all and re-spooled them one by one until you and the world made sense to each other. I won't say 'again' because I think it was new to you.

You were always stubborn. And although I admire people who won't and don't give up, sometimes I felt you were as blind to courage as you were to laughter, and so blind to disaster. You who used to chuckle in your sleep.

What I'm trying to say is there is the big picture and there are the dots; and often, it is the dots that sustain us. Celestial fireflies.

Make your own light and light your own path – be guided by what you know is right and never just by what others say.

There is no such thing as 'I can't help it'. We all have a choice, and we always have a choice. Even the Japanese prisoner condemned to die to test the famous diagonal cut of a new Samurai sword tempered for decades by a master craftsman, even that poor wretch got the last laugh by swallowing stones on the eve of his execution.

Each in his own way can say: 'Let there be light!'

Or peck at everything like a hen pecking at your brain. Peck it apart or let it be.

It has been said that 'If you frighten people enough, you can make them do anything'. And that is why we have to fight fear. Coraggio! I wanted to fight your battles for you, but that doesn't work. You knew that before I did, so you battled your demons alone.

And now you have the power and you have distilled it into words.

I wish I had the words to tell you how proud I am of you.

*Mamma*

# Author's Note

The mental health unit I was admitted to forms part of Wonford House, which first opened its doors on 7<sup>th</sup> July 1869 as a 'hospital for the insane'. No doubt, much has changed since then but the daunting facade of that big Victorian manor has not. The first time I saw it I was in the back of an ambulance thinking what a good start to a horror movie it would make.

My ward was Delderfield and inside its walls, behind its locked blue doors, were some of the most extraordinary people I've ever met. One of them (a fellow patient) told me a story about Vincent Van Gogh, an urban legend that tells how the artist believed that eating his yellow oil paint would help him become happier. I didn't know whether the story was true, but I did know what it meant to want to change your inner state so much that you'd try anything.

What follows are the poems I started writing on the ward.

"...Florence appeared well kempt. Normal rate, tone and volume of speech. Mood was subjectively and objectively euthymic. She still described ongoing intrusive thoughts and mentioned using bulimia as a way of self-medicating but was starting to take control of it. Not thought disordered, no delusions or perceptual abnormality. Florence had insight and was future oriented.

Florence continued to improve on the ward and was eating well. She also confirmed being better and also able to write more poems on the ward as she has not been able to do that previously.

Florence was engaging well in OT activities, polite in interaction with both staff and peers.

She also started psychotherapy while on the ward."

*Discharge Summary*
*Delderfield Ward, The Cedars*

# EATING YELLOW

# Delderfield

There's a sign in the entrance hall,
In front of a locked blue door;
It says 'WELCOME'.
Well, at least it used to.
The 'L' is missing.
Its outline, marked in dust.
Now it says 'WE COME'.
There are stains on the ceiling,
Brown like old blood.
Like a single serving
Of decaf espresso,
Thrown from a paper cup.
Everything has buttons:
The thermos,
The shower,
The patients,
The taps.
And if you press the wrong ones,
Nothing at all comes out
Or everything all at once.

There's a sound to listen for;
The sound is key,
It's the sound of the door
Unlocking.
A hushed 'tick'
And for a second it clicks open,
Then quickly,
Quietly,
Shut.
Damn!
I think I missed it...

Wait by the blue door,
Stare through the glass,
The smears and fingerprints.
The screws on the handle are loose:
Overuse and frustration.
From behind the door
You wait and you listen.
Listen for the sound of footsteps on the floor:
The right kind, mind you,
The right kind are key.
I'm listening;
Trying to hear over the rants
That ebb and flow inside.
Above the shouting man in the purple chair
Who says 'Listen!' 'LISTEN!'
To no one there.
It's not the steps of socked feet.
Not restless, pacing trainers.
Not the dragging kind in slippers.
No.
Nurses' steps sound different.
Their uniforms swish with purpose: jingle with keys.
Finally, the door is open.
I wonder when we get to leave.

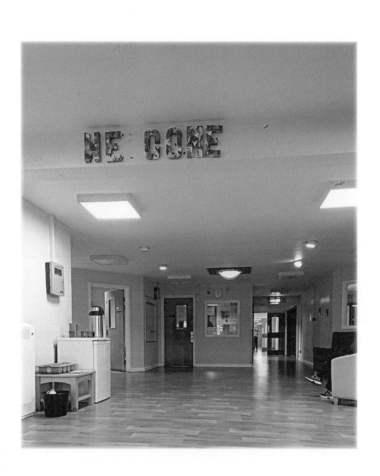

## All's Quiet in Coombehaven

My room's number 7,
It has no desk and no curtain,
But the window has a view
Of a little courtyard garden.
I press my forehead to the metal mesh
I'm a mosquito,
Feeling my way for a hole in the net.
There are flowers
Like the ones you used to wear;
It's a little piece of heaven
But I'm not allowed in there.
That's only for Coombehaven,
That's only for downstairs.

So I watch through the window.
Aladdin's playing solitaire,
The wind smokes his cigarette.
He's going to join the Navy soon,
When he's better, he says...
I think of them downstairs,
On their bean bags,
On their beds.
Turning up their headphones,
Shaking their heads.
A shouting voice
Sounds like any other,
Becomes someone's father, brother.
A woman's scream
Reminds a man downstairs of mother.
Mother...

But someone else was happy here:
Someone before.
There's a smiley face scribbled on my door.
On the white board you can still read two lines:
They say 'fix my mind'
And 'mother is a swine'.
Permanent marker...
Lasts longer than you'd think.

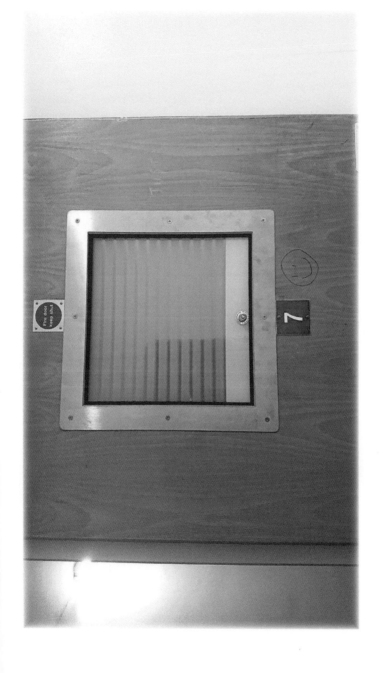

# Requiem for a Television

One morning the TV went quiet:
Dead.
The news anchor
Was killed off
Mid-sentence,
No warning:
I'll never know what he said.
All the colour in existence
Went missing,
Zapped out.
It's nothing to clap about.
Now all that is left is... Us.


Now *we* are the shadow figures,
The ones who haunt the fish tank.
The insanity
That stares back
With your own eyes.
Sad, shuffling visitors,
Protagonists of a darkened dream.
All the madness in the room
Reflected,
Playing out, onscreen.
Black mirror prisoners:
We're the ghosts in the machine.

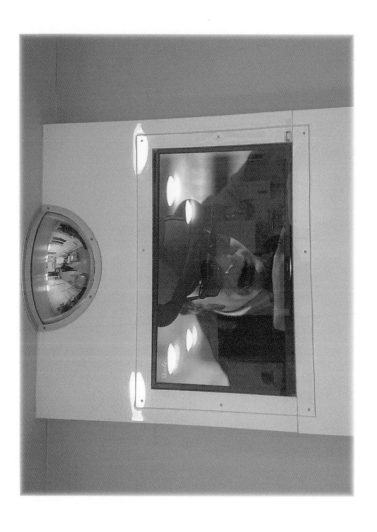

## Just Another Fruit in the Bowl

The wellies were a mistake.
The others don't like them.
I've been accused
Of being a farmer,
Asked
If I'm expecting a flood.
   Never mind,
   Things are looking up!
The thermos is out
For the first time this week,
(It's been sequestered
In the nurses' station.)
Someone had used it inappropriately,
It had to be removed,
That was the official explanation.
He's at it again, look!
Rearranging the fruit
Into a sort of tower.
He's waiting for the moment
Someone chooses an orange;
A banana rolls...
And the whole thing plummets
Back into the fruit bowl.

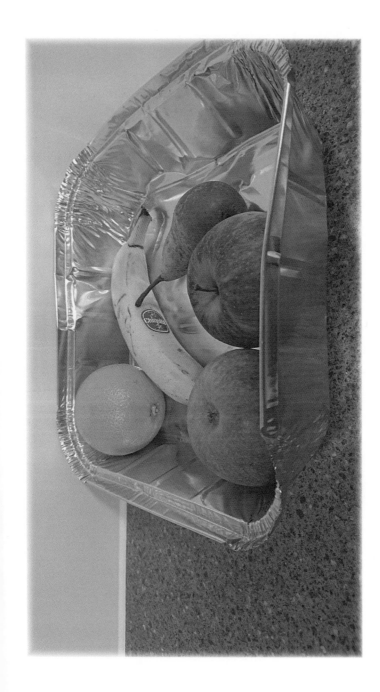

## What Kind of Hospital is This?

Word on the ward is
She's a published author:
A poet.
Listens to the news in French,
Prefers to eat alone,
Speaks foreign languages.
She thinks there's someone in the ceiling,
Sometimes she can hear them speaking;
I think we're friends.

While the ward's asleep
She writes things on the doctor's door...
'What kind of hospital is this?'
All along the white-washed walls,
They keep being repainted.
It's an ongoing battle
That quietly rages
Between a painter with his roller
And a poet with her mighty pen.
He's got no chance
In his overalls,
He'll be back again.

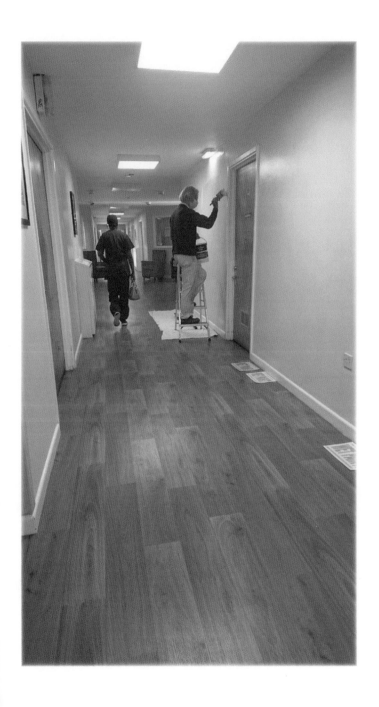

# The Restless Wordsmith

His legs won't stop shaking,
He bounces tables on his knee.
Now my food's vibrating,
Fish fillet's heading for the peas.
Something to do with medication;
Can't quite remember now
ADHD...?

We have Phish Food for pudding,
That's a flavour of ice cream,
(He explains to the confused face
of the cook in the canteen).

There he is,
Have you seen?
The restless Wordsmith,
The soldier,
The joker,
The artist.
A bit of this,
A mix of that,
A touch of paranoid psychosis...

He talks like someone pressed fast forward;
Stock exchange,
Crypto,
The political climate.
He's a humming neon light,
Loud and bright,
Switched on all the time.

There he is,
Can you see him?
High above the 'averages',
Bouncing off the walls
With his tattoos and his bandages.
A free-thinking mind
Full of thoughts and nightmares:
Van Gogh,
Red Square,
Rainbow pythons.

When he's not being chased by terrorists
He breakfasts on Amphetamines,
Feeds his snakes microwaved mouse.
He's too fast paced for *this* place,
They can't keep up with his mouth.
And words are like locks here:
A way in
And a way out,
Better than a locksmith...
In a madhouse.

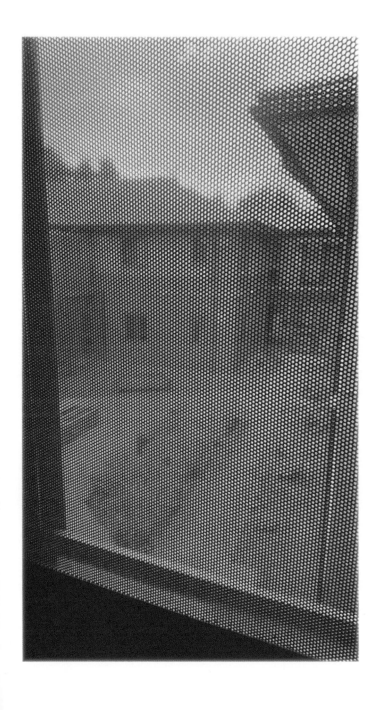

## Mandy's Got a Visitor

Mandy's got a visitor,
He's been loitering about
Since this morning,
Asking after her.
He's had a rollie off me
And 2 papers,
I told him Mandy's not awake yet
She gets up... later.
"Ello darlin'!' She says when she sees him.
They don't hug.
Or even seem to touch,
Just circle each other
Like two planets in orbit,
Following their own gravitational laws.
They sit very close
Sharing a bubble of smoke,
He doesn't say very much,
Then again,
He doesn't have to.
"Ear, I got a joke for you.'
She tells him
Ashing on his trainers.
He looks like he could do with a joke
Like he hasn't laughed in ages...
'A patient goes to see Dr Turner, says can you 'elp me? I'm
addicted to Twitter.'
'What? Sorry I don't follow you!'
He doesn't react at all.
Maybe he's heard better,

Or heard that one before
Along with all the others.
The bullfrog with the five legs,
What's worse than a Tory government?
Etcetera etcetera...
He plays Bob Dylan on his phone,
Her favourite.
The sound is crackling
Speaker's a bit broken.
But she sings along,
He smiles, and for a moment...
Who'd have thought it?
Now they are just one planet, in orbit.

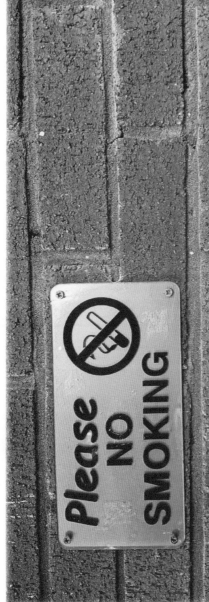

# Nicotine and Rain

The cigarette butts are accumulating
Like ever-sprouting seeds
Along the brick walls of the building,
Under the signs that say
'No Smoking, Please'.
A graveyard of filters stained
by tar and rain.

I think they were meant for planting:
Something living, green.
But weeds *can* be a problem,
They'll take over if you let them...
'Think of all that watering',
Someone must have said,
Never mind the flowers,
Let's do wood chippings instead.

What's left: a toxic soil,
Bark mixed with tobacco.
Dead trees coated
In the ash of other trees
Where filthy papers
Rustle like leaves
And nothing dares to grow,
Not even weeds.

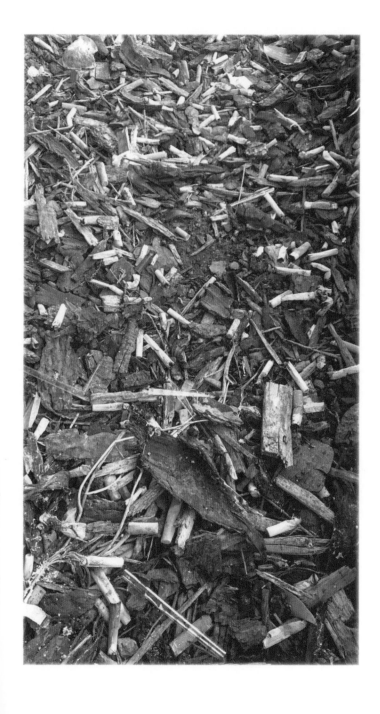

## Ludwell Valley

There are cans of cider in the hedges
And syringes;
Dogs catching frisbees
With their humans,
Kids in the distance
Shooting goals
Into posts without nets.

There's a basketball court
Where the benches are rocks,
My plimsolls are wet with dew,
Soaked right through,
to the socks.

A broken bottle of J20
Is Glistening
On the AstroTurf;
I get a sudden urge
To sweep it up
And buy a basketball...

Told the nurses on the ward
I'd be back before lunchtime
But stay till 'way past'.
I stroke the dogs that come and sniff me,
Warn their humans about the glass.

## Waiting for the Night Staff

The day staff are too tired for another chat, Rich, They've
got lives outside you know:
Pets,
Lovers,
Kids...
The night staff are coming though,
It's nearly time for their shift...


Medusa's worried about her hamster;
In a school play she was a Parrot...
'It's been two weeks
and he's all alone with three slices of carrot!'
She needs to ring her next of kin
But no one's listening...
Places to be,
Places to go.
You'll have to let the night staff know
When they come in.


The farmer asks if she's allowed a basketball.
'I don't see why not'
A day nurse says,
'As long as you're sensible...'
'Double check with the night staff,
though,
I have to go in a minute...'

It's 9 o'clock
and supper isn't out yet.
It's causing an upset.
Someone's kicking newspapers,
Someone needs their meds;
A disorderly queue is forming.
'Can I have water for a cup of tea?'
'A cigarette?'
'Something from the fridge?'
I'm afraid you'll have to wait,
Ten minutes till the change of shift.


'Where's supper?'
'Can you change my bed?'
'What about my hamster...?'
Two nurses cross gazes:
Hang in there,
They seem to say,
The night staff are coming,
They're on their way.

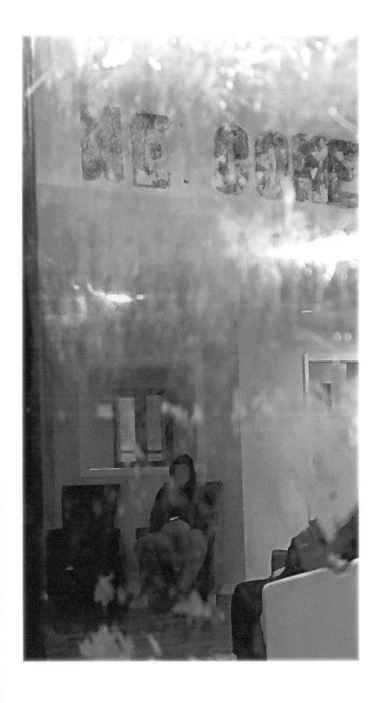

## Channelling Tracy at Lunchtime

I want to be really old,
Stop shaving.
Dye my hair pink,
Maybe red...
Wear age inappropriate clothing.
Never care what anybody thinks,
Or says,
Like Tracy.
I want to raise some eyebrows
To new and dangerous heights,
Cause a scene,
Make a bit of a fuss.
Start fights with people I don't know,
Don't like,
For no good reason.
That sort of stuff.


I want to come home
On my motorbike
In the middle of the night,
Wake up the whole street.
Get the curtain-twitching neighbours
Shouting,
Their dogs and cats and goldfish barking:
I want someone to ring the police.
Want to trip up a jogger,
Wearing high vis.
Sky blue eye shadow,
My whole jewellery box
On my wrists...

I want to be draped
In furry things.
Just to piss off
All the vegans.
Open my car door
Right into a cyclist.

Chain-smoke cigarettes
Smothered in red lipstick,
So every ashtray I ever came across
Looked like it had a period.
I want to smoke while I eat on the toilet
And during sex,
Want smoke to follow me around
Like second breath.
Stub one out in someone else's
Fried egg, at the cafe,
Order a platter of biscuits
And goose liver pate
With an extra plate...
For my dog.

I want all the people
Who ever said:
'I'll drop round soon as I can'
But never did,
To be buried somewhere;
Their bodies
Dismembered and scattered
Over a vast rural area.
I want to be absent
At all of their funerals
And send no flowers.
Sip brandy in my garden shed,

Tending to my crop
Of hydroponic marijuana.
Listening to Ariana Grande
In Hello Kitty pyjamas.

Next door's got a file on me.
There's a folder on her PC
With my name on it.
She's the sort that writes letters.
Got a policeman for a cousin.
Someone'll take care of her
I reckon...
She's got her eye on me,
Likes to spy on me
Through a gap
In the garden gate;
But I slept with her husband.
Twice.
She should write about that,
Put that in her little 'formal complaint'...

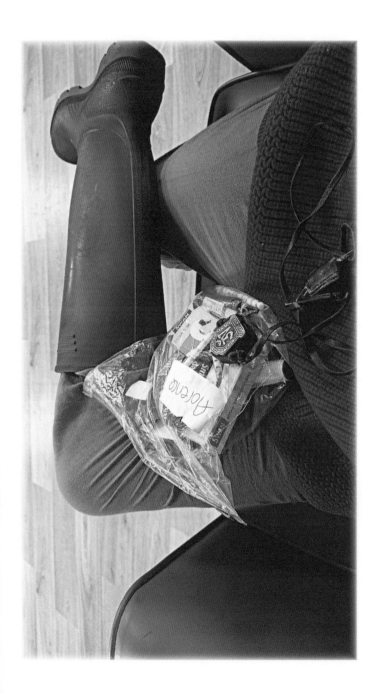

## Death Threats to the Convent

The hand that holds the dagger
Has been slightly...
   *Adjusted.*
To better fit the current...
   *Sentiment.*
These are volatile times:
Unprecedented.
And well,
The dagger,
You see was...
Simply too...
   *Offensive!*
Yes, people were upset.
They protested.
The convent received
Death threats!
Now 'The Last Supper' is
Well... Better!
Do you see?
*Now,* Judas leans into Mary Magdalene
Concealing nothing more than...
A Pomegranate.

## Eat Properly

Life is a blessing.
A gift.
An STD.
Eat your childhood trauma,
Post-traumatic stress disorder.
Stash a chicken carcass
Under your mattress,
Gorge on the rotting flesh.
Eat your feelings,
Your stress,
The Mercury in tuna.
Save the planet
And the flora:
Eat the people,
Not the fauna.
Drink the Fluoride in the water.
Eat your Teflon.
Kindergarten Radon.
Eat your five a day,
Your vegetables,
Monsanto chemicals,
Slaughterhouse spoils,
Supermarket horse.
Eat organic tomatoes
From Phillip Morris soil:
Eat the cancer
In your pasta sauce.
Meditation is a YouTube video.
Sleep is an App.

Eat the Antrax
In the baby food,
Eat your yoga mat.
Consume the ads,
Swallow the narrative,
Follow the yellow brick road.
Eat the carrot,
The stick,
The rabbit and the hole.
Eat the vaccine,
Eat the protests,
Pay your taxes.
Eat your placards,
Eat the anti-vaxxers.
Scroll through the Amazon,
Hang the Orangutans!
Save the palm oil,
Beat the virus,
Kill the bat.
Eat your antidepressants,
Greenhouse gases,
Blow on the planet: eat that!
Eat your rovers
And rockets,
Electric cars,
Reduce your calorie intake
And carbon emissions.
Make greener decisions:
Eat life on Mars.
Eat the debt,
The war chest,

Your contribution.
Eat the food stamps,
Benefits and brollies:
Eat the Revolution.
Eat your happy pills,
Happy meals,
Maladaptive coping skills:
Eat your Russian dollies.
Binge on the shame
Of fast fashion,
Black Friday sales,
The heavy metals in the rain:
Eat the chemtrails.
Feed the children,
The pollution,
Ingest the pain.
Starve yourself
For the vanity fair,
Be a corporate victim;
Airbrushed,
Catwalk mannequin.
Eat your heart out,
Double-tap the heart-shaped box.
Eat the photo filters,
The Emojis,
Eat the botox.
Stay hungry:
Eat nothing.
Pick the foam from your armchair,
Eat the stuffing.
Help yourself

To another dumpling,
Another scoop,
Another dollop.
Now kneel down,
Bow your head:
Vomit.
Paint the inside of the toilet
Like a Jackson Pollock.
Feel the high,
The emotional release,
Never mind
The organ damage.
Purge the dark thoughts
That your mind spawned
Like your mouth
had a miscarriage.
Eat your suicidal thoughts,
Your eating disorder,
The payoffs, the chaos,
Eat the 'New World Order'.
Eat your face mask
And finish your Broccoli.
People are starving.
Eat properly.

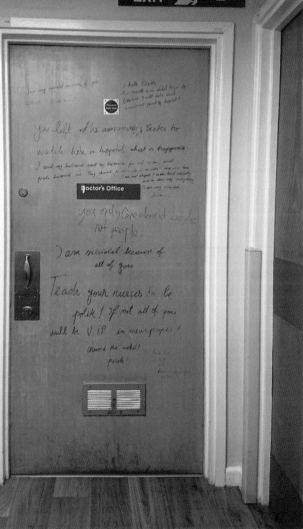

## No Doctor, Yes Doctor, But

The TV's communicating
With me,
And it's got a really bad message.
No doctor,
I'm not schizophrenic.
Yes doctor,
Still taking the antidepressants...
But doctor!
The Apps on my phone
Want all sorts of access,
And I'm worried that one day
My mattress
Will be able to record our dreams
And send the live stream to Davos.
No doctor,
I can't always stomach the chaos.
Yes, Doctor, I know
That I need to keep eating.

But doctor!
What about the ghosts I drove through?
They were crossing the roads
On the way to Maputo.
Then the electric fan
Became a desert man...
But do *you* know why he was dancing a tango?
And doctor, how do you explain
That gnome at my window:
The one who let in the spiders?
Or the ivy that sprawled
Across the whole floor,
When my bedroom turned into a garden...

I know doctor, you don't know.
So why are we here splitting hairs?
Doctor, I've seen what it looks like
Behind all the layers!
The carpets are breathing,
The statues are bleeding,
And no doctor, no,
I haven't been sleeping.

## Cutting Teeth

Beware the machine man
And his iron-tasting kisses:
He'll chew the inside of your cheeks
Before you even know you're bitten.
He's the chip in your enamel
You cut your tongue to smooth,
You probe him like a cavity
But you're not searching for the truth.

He's the white-coat knee
Pressing on your chest
With a sharp tool
And a doll house mirror.
He's the panic in your stomach
After waking
From a toothless nightmare.

A wisdom tooth
That cut too crooked:
His name on your breath
Like a dry socket.
The bloodied bite mark
In a piece of fruit,
You'd fracture your own jaw
To pull out his roots.

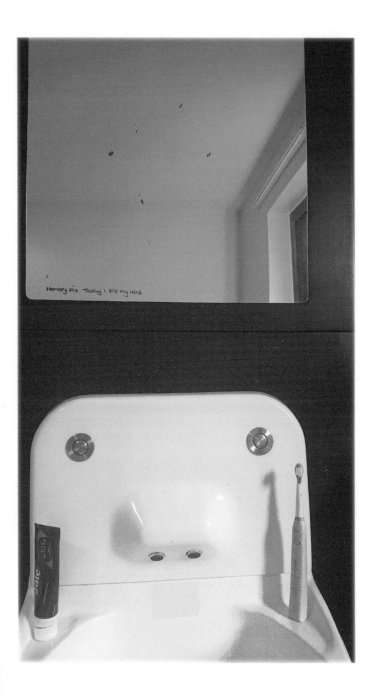

# Hate, Dreams and Answering Machines

I can write about anything:
Hate,
Dreams.
Answering machines,
Anything but you.
If there are words to describe you,
I don't know them,
I wasn't taught them in school.

You make my other poems pointless:
You're the best lines I'll never use.
Asked my parents for the words once,
They made them up.
I knew they weren't the right ones,
But they sounded close enough.
And I thought that love would teach me,
Ease the words out like a splinter;
But love just placed a kiss there,
Let the skin grow over.

Hate became my last hope,
Invited me to its talk show,
So of course, I went.
I hung the dirty washing on the line:
Yours and mine,
Hate handed me the pegs.
The audience clapped
While the spin doctors sighed
And nothing very nice was said...

Hate promised it would stay in touch
But now it's busy, going 'ghost'.
Keeps leaving me on 'read',
Never 'likes' my posts.
Again last night,
You gatecrashed
One of my better dreams...
I think I may have left hate a message
On your answering machine.

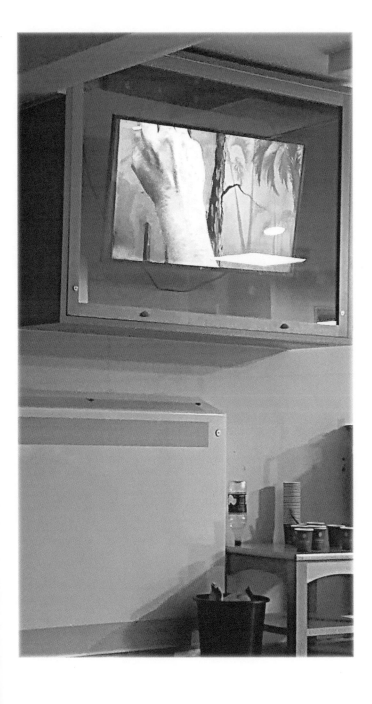

## Rainy Day in Slough

The devil stuck a straw in the sky,
Sucked all the Blue Curaçao,
Snorted the chemtrails,
Got high ...
Now it's probably raining in Slough.
There are tears
In the gravy on Sunday,
A spin cycle cackles
In the basement.
A storm brews in an ashtray,
The rain flicks its butts
On the pavement.
There's puddle water in the syringes,
Rain lands on cracked hands
And splinters,
Thunder coughs in the distance,
Lightning strikes in the vein.
Dreaming of being a rare plant
In Kew Gardens, just for an hour,
Blissed out until I remember:
They'll probably kill me
When I don't flower.

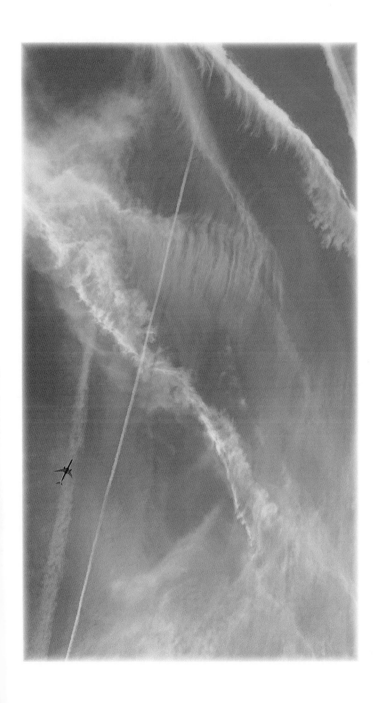

## Chelsea Embankment

Letting go
Is like trying to pack
Everything you ever had
Into a piece of hand luggage:
The size may look right at the desk,
But the weight is massive.
Yes, it will fit into the overhead compartment.
No, It won't bring down the plane.
But where's that ballerina from my music box?
Where's the way that you used to say my name?
I bet she doesn't pirouette to Chopin any more,
Who could blame her?
I hope that someone finds her in a thrift store
Or a landfill, somewhere...


Letting go
Is like walking away
With a suitcase that's missing a wheel.
A 'bag for life' with a hole,
Chewing gum holding a heel.
Yes, it's prettier from the Embankment
But it won't move the city to rain.
Where's the ring that slipped under the floorboards?
Where's the spirit of the woman who came?
Now she's buried in a graveyard, somewhere,
But the pier looks much the same.
I wonder if someone is bringing her flowers;
If the river remembers her name.

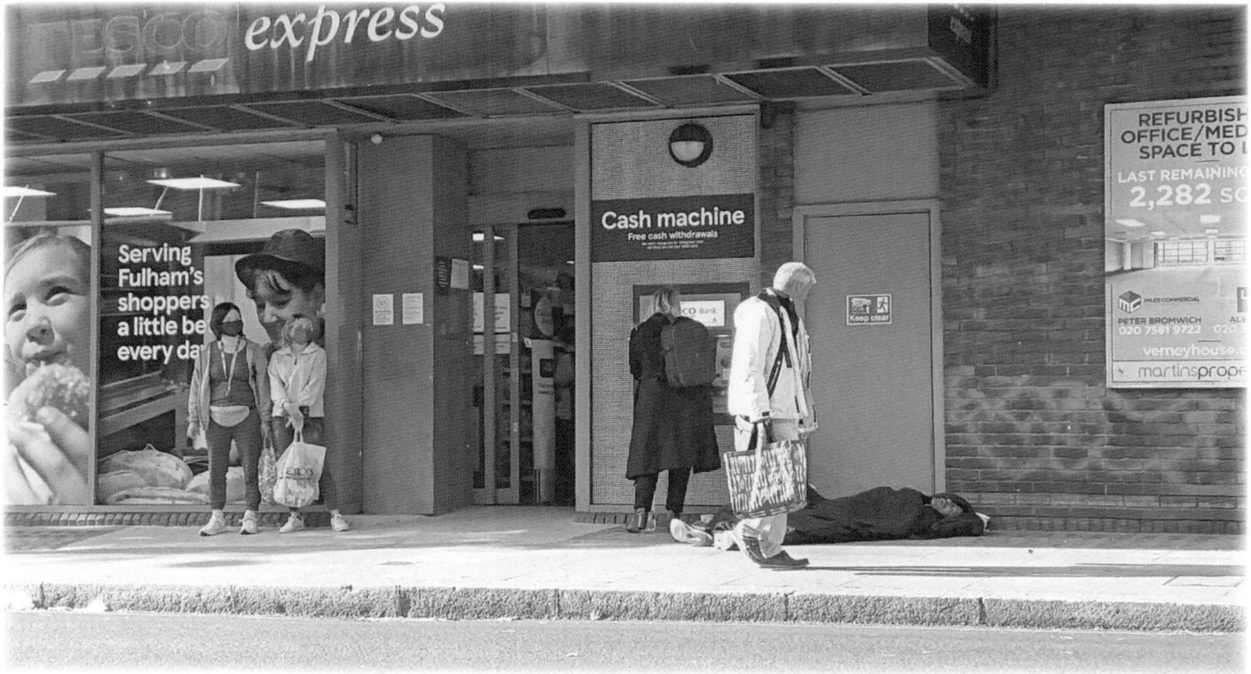
express
Cash machine
Free cash withdrawals
Serving
Fulham's
shoppers
Keep clear
2,282
PETER BROMWICH
020 7581 9722

## Silent Whistle

Press your ear to the pulse of the past:
Sounds like a train that just passed.
Sounds like the tail end of some distant laugh,
The thud of a rock being dropped
On a bird in the grass.
Do not trespass, there be dragons!
There'll be maggots in the entrails;
Every chair you try to sit on
Has a woodworm in the crossrail.
The orchard's full of fruit,
But there's a wasp in every plum;
With every bite,
You move your mouth
To being stung.


Cup my hand to the shell of my ear:
Sounds like a shipwreck is near.
Storm crows are already here,
They're sinking my dreams in the tide...
      *No.*
   *It's just a storm outside...*
Cracking down on the willow;
But I'm thinking that I'd like to drown
In the sweat on your pillow.

Press your ear to the pulse of the past:
Sounds like the sea making glass.

Lifting a veil, giving head.
The hiss of a dress unzipped,
Kicked to the foot of the bed.
Warm trembling lips
Kissing the cheeks of the dead.
Sounds like the hollow
You lay down your armour to follow.
Shed your teeth in the mirror,
Lose your locks in the bristles;
We come when it calls,
It's the silent whistle.

# Return to Mother (ama-gi)

Let me be born,
Deep in a forest,
Somewhere.
No white light,
No scalpel,
No forceps.
Let me crawl to the breast of my mother;
Her skin is my cover.
I've not been cold before.


My lungs will fill
For the first time
With cool wind and pollen,
My cry will startle a robin...
　　Karma hasn't forgotten
　　What I have to give,
But let me live.
Deep in a forest
Somewhere...
No rental,
No cottage,
No villa.
Let me roam,
The woods are my shelter.
I won't be cold for long.

The oak and the ash are my walls,
Moss is my memory foam.
Stars on the ceiling,
Embers on the floor,
My pillow's all bluebells and thunder!
I'll listen to the fire
As it slips into the choir of nocturnal hunters.

Skylarks, wake me at dawn!
My breakfast's a marmalade sunrise.
I'll run through the trees
Until my skin is warm,
Wash the ghosts from my mind in the river...

Let me be buried,
Deep in a forest,
Somewhere.
No gravestone.
No coffin.
No scripture.
Bury me naked;
The earth is my blanket,
I'll never be cold again.

Let the maggots grow fat on my eyes,
Mushroom spores colonise
And spread like veins in the dark:
They are my lungs and my heart.

With worms in my nostrils,
My scars are blackberry brambles.
No debt in my pockets,
No pennies on my eyelids,
No shackles.
The cuffs round my ankles
Are daisy chains now,
My worries are wild sage.
Toadstools hatch over my bones,
Daffodils root in my ribcage.

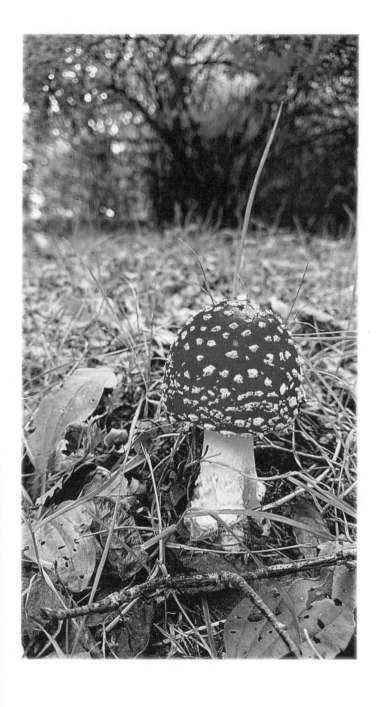

# About Florence Duff-Scott

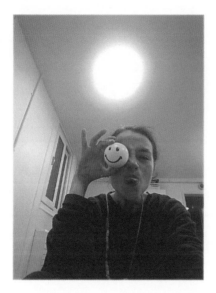

On the day this picture was taken, I was in a temporary facility on the outskirts of London, waiting for the next available bed in a mental health unit. I was tired: tired in that way that doesn't let you sleep, the tiredness of someone who's been trying to keep their head above water for so long that they have no fight left. After having felt so numb inside, I found myself ambushed by every emotion I'd ever suppressed. With a vengeance, every feeling I'd buried came flooding up, and like a burst dam, the tears I hadn't let myself cry, poured out.

There was a nurse at the facility assigned the task of watching over me. He made many attempts to calm and comfort me but I couldn't hear him. Sunken to that place inside myself where tears replace words, his kindness couldn't reach me. That is until he crouched beside me and offered me a yellow ball, a stress ball which smiled up at me from the palm of his hand. My first thought when I saw it was that my daughter would love it and I imagined her cheeky smile. In that moment, a little brightness returned, a glimmer of yellow; her face in my mind's eye like sunlight dancing on the surface.

That day I sent her this photo with a promise: I promised that when I was feeling better, the yellow ball would be hers, and now it is.

In aid of

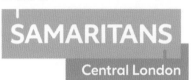

Central London Samaritans, based in the heart of London, is the founding branch of the wider Samaritans organisation. Our volunteers provide confidential, non-judgemental, emotional support to anyone who is struggling to cope for whatever reason. Anyone can contact Samaritans FREE any time from any phone (even a mobile without credit) on:

## 116 123

This number won't show up on your phone bill.

We're here to listen every hour of every day, and have provided this support without interruption since opening in 1953 at St Stephen Walbrook. We respond to around 70,000 requests for help each year via phone calls, email and webchat, as well as taking our services to vulnerable individuals at highest risk of suicide, such as homeless people, people in prison, people in custody and those bereaved by suicide.

In June 2022, we reopened our doors to face-to-face visitors. Anyone can come to our branch every day from 9am to 9pm with no appointment or referral. We're delighted to be providing this service again; after all, face-to-face support is how Samaritans first began 70 years ago.

Every call we answer could be the one that saves or changes someone's life – the call that ends with someone finding the strength to keep going.

**www.samaritans.org**

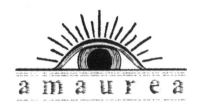

amaurea

**More poetry published by Amaurea Press:**

Anna Lidia Vega Serova, *Un Jardín en Minatura/A Garden in Miniature* (poems, with photographs by Gonzalo Vidal)

Combining poetry and photography, a bilingual (Spanish and English) edition, in which text and image are brought together in poetic conversation. The poems deal with love and loss, hybrid identity, and the planting of our dreams in the midst of urban decay.

Hardback, 124pp., with colour photographs
ISBN 978-010914278-00-6

Anna Lidia Vega Serova, *Sideways Glance*

A book about the most everyday of objects, bringing together the fragments of a life, outlines that become confessions or discoveries. Anna Lidia presents a vision of the surrounding world through the briefest of glances – playing, always playing.

Paperback 124pp., with black and white drawings
ISBN 978-010914278-02-0

For further details about these and other Amaurea publications, visit www.amaurea.co.uk

Printed in Great Britain
by Amazon

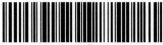

29569422R00059

ISBN 9798645626662

9 798645 626662